Fall Prevention:
Stay On Your Own Two Feet!

Second Edition

Fall Prevention Advisors, LLC
Gail Davies, PT, MS,GCS
Fran Scully, PT
Illustrations by Pam Gosner

ISBN 0-7414-3239-0

Published by:

INFINITY
PUBLISHING.COM
1094 New DeHaven Street, Suite 100
West Conshohocken, PA 19428-2713
Info@buybooksontheweb.com
www.buybooksontheweb.com
Toll-free (877) BUY BOOK
Local Phone (610) 941-9999
Fax (610) 941-9959

Printed in the United States of America
Printed on Recycled Paper
Published September 2008

Dedicated to the memory of
Robert Stenard Sr. and
Thomas and Frances Marinaccio

Introduction

Falls and fear of falling are a major challenge to living independently.
- One in three people over the age of 65 (living in the community) will fall during the next year.
- Hip fractures are common fall injuries that can cause a loss of independence and lead to nursing home placement.
- Falls are the leading cause of death from injury in people age 65 or over.

Strength and balance exercises can reduce your risk of a fall.
- Balance and strength can be improved with exercise.
- Practicing Tai Chi improves balance.
- Regardless of age, strength training increases muscle mass.
- Studies have shown 90 year olds will increase their strength with exercise.

We have been physical therapist for over twenty years and were motivated to write fall prevention books after treating many patients with fall related injuries.

A comprehensive fall prevention program needs to reduce fall risk factors by addressing home safety, physical well being (vision, medications, shoes, etc) and life situation.

Information and statistics taken from AARP, www.aarp.org and CDC, Center for Disease Control www.cdc.gov.

About The Authors and Illustrator

Gail Davies has over 20 years experience as a physical therapist and is a board certified geriatric specialist. Her experience is in long term care, private practice and home care.

Fran Scully is also a physical therapist. She has worked primarily in rehabilitation, geriatrics and long term care.

The authors were motivated to write this book after treating many patients with fall related injuries. They also provide education to care givers and community groups on home modifications and strategies to prevent falls. They can be contacted at www.fallpreventionadvisors.com

Pam Gosner is a professional artist and former children's librarian with many years of experience creating artwork for library programs, as well as illustrating her own books on historic architecture of the West Indies.

Fall Prevention:
Stay On Your Own Two Feet!

Table of Contents

Fall Prevention: Stay On Your Own Two Feet! will raise awareness of common fall hot spots and when to seek appropriate medical intervention. Being informed and proactive can help prevent a trip from becoming a fall. Before starting any exercise program get approval from your physician.

Let's Begin
Stay on Your Own Two Feet!

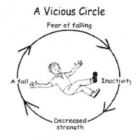

Fear of Falling

A Vicious Circle

A Vicious Circle

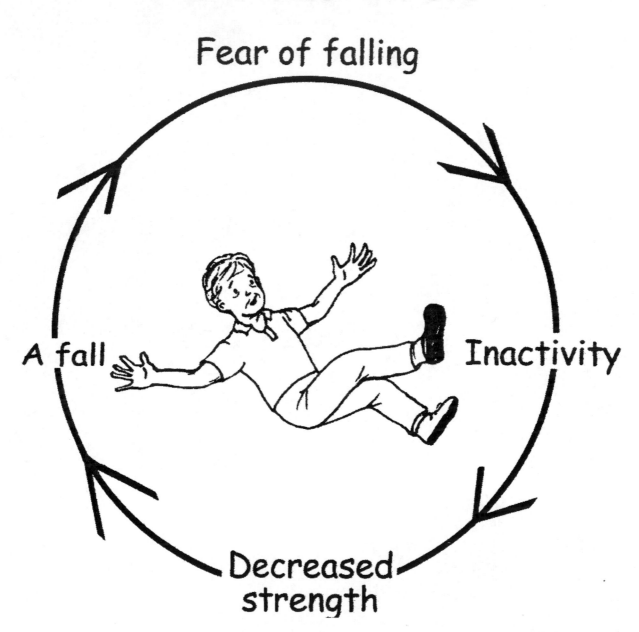

Fear of falling

Inactivity

Decreased strength

A fall

Fear of Falling

Have you/Can you...???
- sit and stand with ease
- had a fall
- ignored a fall because you didn't think it was important
- discussed any falls with your doctor
- curtailed your activity because you are afraid of falling
- stopped exercising because you are afraid of falling
- stopped taking walks because you are afraid of falling
- get up from the floor
- accessible telephones
- heard about fall pendants
- heard about hip protectors

Hot Spot
Fear of Falling

Hot Spots are:
- collapsing into your chair when sitting down
- difficulty standing up from sitting
- ignoring a fall
- not telling your doctor about your fear of falling
- not discussing the circumstances of a fall with your doctor
- not exercising
- no accessible telephones
- limiting activity due to fear of falling
- fear of not being able to get up from the floor

**Inactivity is not the answer to preventing falls.
Inactivity can actually cause a fall!**

A vicious circle develops...
- ➢ the fear of falling leads to inactivity
- ➢ inactivity leads to increased weakness
- ➢ weakness leads to a fall
- ➢ the fall increases the fear of falling
- ➢ the fear of falling leads to inactivity

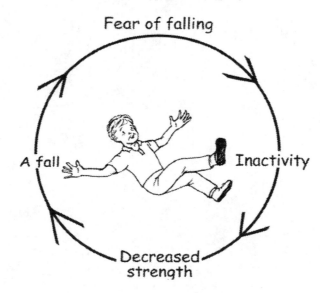

A Vicious Circle

Fear of falling

A fall

Inactivity

Decreased strength

Solutions for Fear of Falling

Know how to sit with ease...and not "fall" into your chair

- back up to the chair so you feel it behind your knees
- reach back and hold armrests or seat with your hands
- bend at your waist and knees
- lead with your buttocks
- gracefully sit down

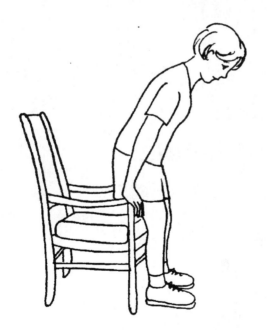 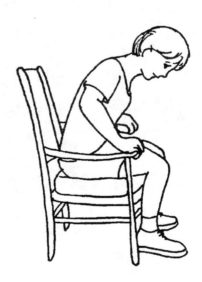

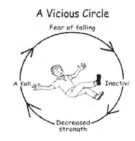

A Vicious Circle

Know how to stand with ease...
- scoot to edge of chair/couch
- slide feet back, slightly behind knees and apart
- place hands on arm rests if available, or on seat
- lean forward over your knees
- push up on the armrests shifting weight forward over your feet, stand
- if you are lightheaded when first standing wait before walking until you feel steady, discuss this lightheadedness with your doctor as it can often be treated

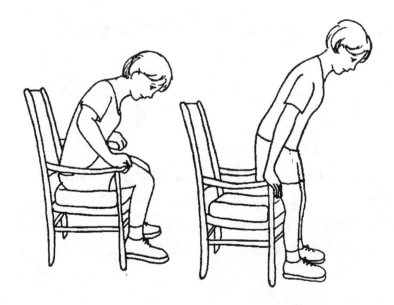

Solutions for Fear of Falling

See your doctor
- rule out any medical cause for fear of falling
- review all medications and their side effects
- discuss benefits of strength/balance/Tai Chi program
- get approval for participating in an exercise program
- get referral for physical therapist for treatment or to design home exercise program specific to your needs

If you have fallen discuss the following with your doctor...
- how you fell
- the time of day
- where you were
- what you were doing
- what shoes/clothing you were wearing
- what you thought the cause was
- what medications you had taken
- and of course any pain or injury from the fall
- fear of falling

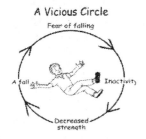

A Vicious Circle

Start your exercise program! (with your doctor's approval)
There are many options available. The goal is to safely
increase your activity level.
- start by reading the sections on strength, balance,
  posture and you will learn that exercise can help
  prevent falls
- start a walking program/join a mall walking program
- see a physical therapist for treatment of more involved
  balance/strength/posture problems and obtain an
  exercise program
- call your local Area Agency on Aging for fall prevention
  exercise programs in your area

**Telephones need to be accessible from the floor in the
event of a fall.**
- Telephones should be located in all of the most
  frequently used rooms, including the bathroom,
  basement, laundry room or get in the habit of bringing
  a cordless or cell phone with you as you move about.
- Multi-pack phones require only one phone jack for the
  main phone and come with other phones that only
  need to be plugged into an electrical outlet to work.

Solutions for Fear of Falling

Know how to get up from the floor. This will help prevent panicking in the event of a fall.

Read the following instructions.

Look at the pictures on the next page.

- Move/crawl/scoot along floor to a large stable piece of furniture. A low piece of furniture will provide the best support to help you get up.
- When in front of furniture get on your hands and knees.
- Place hands on furniture. (If the chair seat is too high you can always put your hands under the cushions.)
- Place one foot flat on floor and curl the toes on the other foot so they are gripping the floor.
- Using your arm and legs push up and stand.
- Sit on chair/couch.

In the event of a fall the first step is to relax and take inventory to see if you are injured and then to use your accessible phone or fall pendant to summon help.

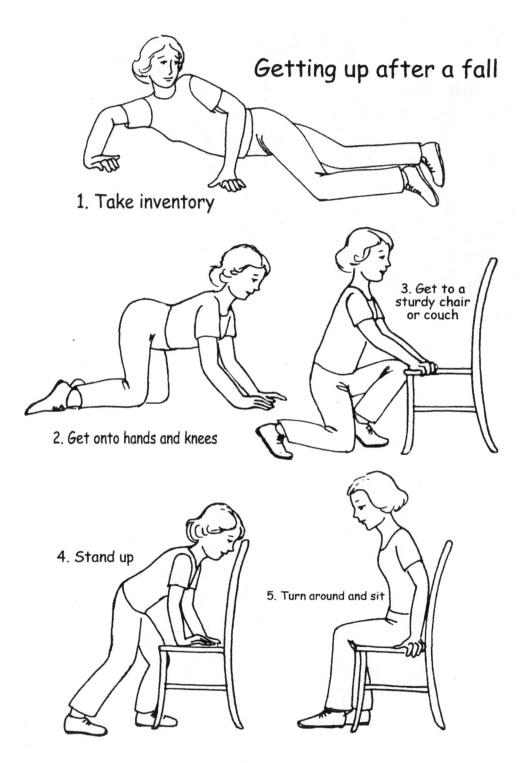

Getting up after a fall

1. Take inventory

2. Get onto hands and knees

3. Get to a sturdy chair or couch

4. Stand up

5. Turn around and sit

Devices to ease fear of falling.

Fall Pendants:
- provide security
- can be worn on the wrist, around the neck, or clips on a belt, they should be water proof and worn in the shower/bath
- when activated it notifies a response center who then contacts a pre-designated doctor, family member or friend
- some companies that supply pendants include:
    American Medical Alarms 1 800 542-0438
    Philips Lifeline 1 800 380-3111
    Medical Alert Alarm System 1 800 906 0872
    Life Alert 1 800 815-5922
- also contact the Red Cross, or local Senior Citizen Center as they can provide information on cost and how to buy/rent a fall pendant in your area.

Hip Protectors.
If you and your doctor decide you are considered high risk for a fall you may want to try wearing hip protectors. They are clothing with hip pads to help minimize hip injury from a fall. Available through surgical supply stores and catalogs.

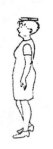

Posture

Stand Tall

Stand Tall

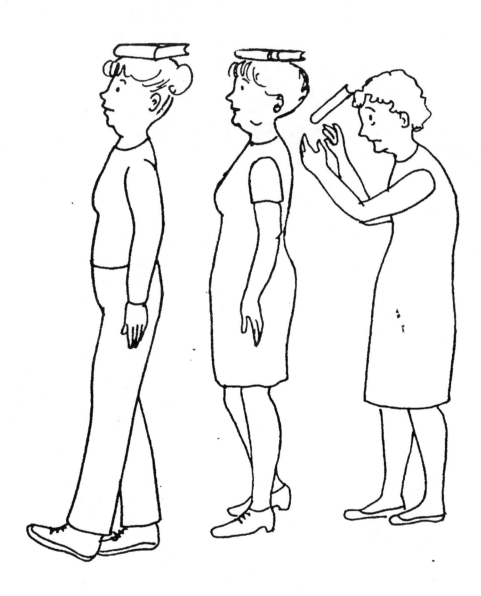

Posture

Do you/Have you???

- have poor posture
- have osteoporosis
- had a bone density test
- stand tall and not slouch
- do posture exercises
- have good sitting posture
- know how to reach overhead
- know how to bend and lift

Hot Spot
Poor Posture

Poor posture can contribute to falls.

Hot spots are:
- neglecting bone health
- posture of forward head and rounded shoulders
- poor standing posture
- not checking/correcting posture habits
- not doing posture exercises
- slouched sitting posture
- incorrect bending and lifting
- incorrectly reaching overhead

Cartoons often show older people bent over. This does not have to happen! Bad habits, osteoporosis and a general loss of strength can contribute to slouched posture. The rounding of the upper back moves our center of gravity forward making it more difficult to maintain balance.

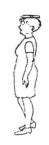

Solutions for Poor Posture

Learn about osteoporosis and how to take care of your bone health.

Osteoporosis occurs when bones lose mass and become thin, brittle and easily broken; particularly the wrist, spine (vertebra) and hip. Osteopenia is the beginning of bone thinning which can progress to osteoporosis if not treated.

- Bone loss can lead to vertebral compression fractures, reduced height, pain in middle/upper back, slumped posture, a hump in the upper back and an increased risk of a fracture from a fall.

  - ❖ Small vertebral (spine) fractures cause a bent over posture.
  - ❖ Balance becomes more difficult to maintain as our center of gravity shifts forward and outside our base of support.

- Have a bone density test.
  - ❖ There is a simple painless test that measures the strength of our bones or bone density.
  - ❖ Women should have a bone density test by age 50. Discuss this test with your doctor.
  - ❖ The results will show if you have any bone loss.

Osteoporosis and Bone Health

- If you have osteoporosis, discuss your exercise plans with your doctor.
    - ❖ Weight bearing exercises are usually recommended to prevent further deterioration of the bones.
    - ❖ See a physical therapist for an exercise program, as there are certain movements that are to be avoided such as bending forward and twisting.

- Discuss changing nutritional needs with your doctor. He may recommend taking calcium supplements/Vitamin D to help build bone mass.

- For more information on osteoporosis we recommend the following books:

    - *Stand Tall, Preventing and Treating Osteoporosis* Morris Notelovitz MD, Ph.D and Diana Tonnessen 1998
    - *Strong Women,Strong Bones* Miriam E. Nelson Ph.D 2000
    - *Walk Tall, An Exercise Program for the Prevention and Treatment of Osteoporosis,* Sara Meeks, PT, G.C.S. 1999
    - *Osteoporosis, An Exercise Guide,* Margie Bessiginger, MS, PT 1998

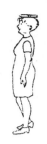

Solution for Poor Posture

Start Posture Exercises: Before doing or starting any exercise program check with your doctor and discuss bone density test results. BUT, you can still have poor posture without having osteopenia or osteoporosis and can benefit from targeted exercises.

- Consider seeing a physical therapist to evaluate <u>your specific needs</u> and to establish an exercise program to improve and protect posture. Establishing a strength training program can help maintain proper body alignment.

- Pilates/core strengthening exercise programs may help improve posture. Pilates exercises focus on strengthening the muscles that keep you upright; abdominal, back and hip muscles.

- A properly designed **yoga** program can increase flexibility and improve posture. There are many different kinds of yoga classes; you are looking for a gentle stretching program. Evaluate the class, see page 39.

A beginning exercise to improve posture is the Chin Tuck.

Chin Tuck Exercise: Do them whenever you think about it, sitting, standing or walking, until it becomes automatic. Pull chin back and squeeze shoulder blades together without lifting your chin or shoulders. Don't hold your breath. You will notice an improvement in your posture.

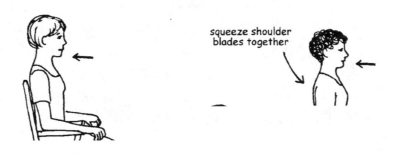

squeeze shoulder blades together

Alison is an accountant who spends her working day over her desk. When trying on dresses for an upcoming wedding she noticed her hunched posture made her look frumpy. She did not like what she saw and this spurred her to contact a physical therapist and start an exercise program to combat and correct her poor posture habits. Within several weeks Alison noticed marked improvement in how she looked and felt.

No doubt you have noticed that people who have good posture look younger.

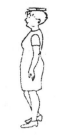

Solution for Poor Posture

Proper Sitting Posture. Slouching while sitting leads to poor posture when standing. Poor posture can contribute to falls.

- Use either a small cushion called a lumbar roll or a back hugger. Available in catalogs/pharmacies.
- A lumbar roll is a small portable cushion that is placed at the small of the back. Both types of cushions discourage a slumped position and helps maintain a correct spine. Below is an illustration of a lumbar roll and a back hugger.

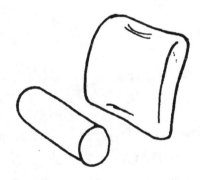

- Proper sitting posture is achieved by having feet flat on the floor with buttocks all the way back until they touch the back of the chair. The lumbar roll is placed at the small of your back and your head is in your "chin tuck position".

- It is useful to place a back hugger in the car/chair to help maintain good posture while driving/sitting.

Use Proper Body Mechanics:

- When bending or lifting use your legs, not your back. This means; bend knees and keep back straight.

- Keeping your feet shoulder width apart creates a wide base of support and improves balance.

- When lifting or carrying items hold them close to your body. Never twist when lifting.

- Carry objects at waist level; don't block your vision.

There can be a tendency to fall backwards when both arms are reaching overhead. To counteract this:

- Stand with feet shoulder width apart and one foot ahead of the other. Maintain this wide base of support for better balance.

- Avoid reaching overhead with both arms at the same time; keep one hand free to hold onto a surface.

- Use a long handle reacher. This handy gadget allows you to reach for an item with one hand either overhead or on the floor. (available in catalogs and stores)

- Rearrange cupboards so all items are within your range of reach. A safe range of reach is approximately an arm's length. Usually, you have to be **taller** than 5'7" to safely reach a top shelf in a kitchen cupboard.

- Use a sturdy step stool with a functional handle; a handle that can be held while standing on the step.

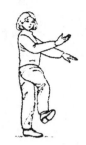

Balance

Improve Your Balance

Improve Your Balance

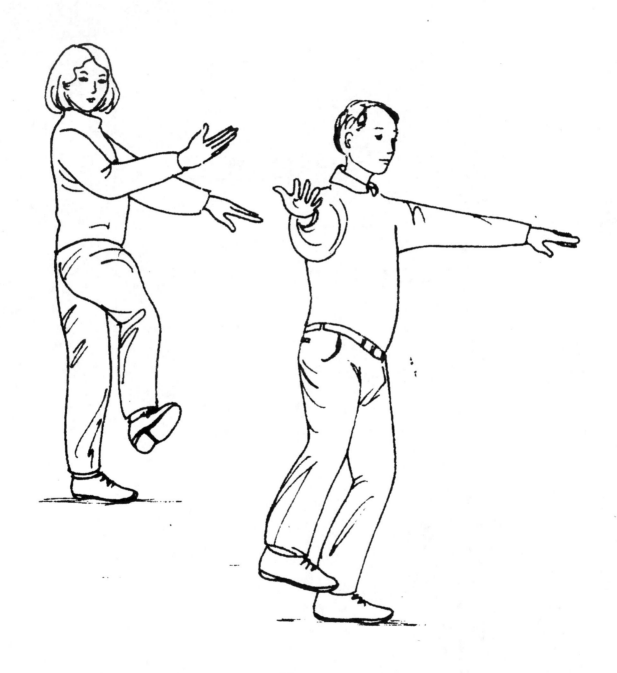

Balance

Do you/Can you???

- stand securely on one leg
- notice changes in balance on thick carpeting
- notice difficulty balancing on outdoor surfaces, such as grass or soft beach sand
- easily carry on a conversation while walking without loss of balance
- take medications on a daily basis
- drink alcohol
- have low blood pressure
- have high blood pressure
- get dizzy when standing up
- have diabetes, arthritis, poor vision, poor posture, Parkinson's disease, or poor circulation

Balance is complex: Three sensory systems, (vision, spatial orientation/proprioception, inner ear) work together along with our muscles to keep us balanced.

Hot Spot
Balance

Without intervention balance starts to decline when we are in our forties.

Hot Spots are:

- sedentary lifestyle
- low or high blood pressure
- light-headedness during changes of position
- room spinning/vertigo*
- racing heart or skipped beats
- colds/ear/sinus infections
- taking medications on a daily basis
- not following correct medication dosage schedule
- sleeping medications
- drinking alcohol
- mixing alcohol and medications
- decreased sensation in feet
- low vision
- limited range of motion
- decreased strength
- impaired reaction time, slower reflexes
- poor posture
- changed walking patterns and pace

*Medical definitions separate dizziness and vertigo. Dizziness is the sensation of unsteadiness or being lightheaded. Vertigo is the sensation of you or the room spinning.

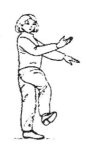

Solutions for Poor Balance

Consult with your doctor:

- **To investigate possible medical causes** for any noticed changes in balance.
- **Discuss existing medical conditions** that may interfere with balance such as arthritis, diabetes, Parkinson's disease, poor vision, poor circulation, cardiovascular disease and osteoporosis. These conditions can restrict range of motion, reduce sensory feedback, impair reaction time and change walking patterns and pace which effects balance.
- Discuss if there is need for an examination and treatment by a physical therapist (PT).
- Discuss the possibility of a referral to a **Balance Assessment Clinic**. Balance Assessment Testing is usually available on an outpatient basis at your local hospital's PT department and can aid your doctor and physical therapist to diagnose, treat and manage vertigo and other balance disorders.
- **Review all medications,** including over the counter, for possible interactions and side effects. Pay special attention to the effects of sleep medications and new prescriptions and how you react to them; some may interfere with balance and alertness.

Solutions for Poor Balance

Consult with your doctor

- **Have your blood pressure checked regularly.** Low and or high blood pressure can cause dizziness.
- **Have your blood pressure checked during position changes.** A drop in blood pressure can sometimes occur with position changes (lying to sitting, sitting to standing) and cause dizziness.
- Do not assume that a **racing heart or skipped beats** are a normal part of aging; irregular heart beats can cause dizziness/faintness and a fall and need to be evaluated by your doctor.
- Ear infections and colds can affect balance. The inner ear is an integral part of our balance system and not to be neglected. See your doctor for treatment of ear problems and don't self treat without medical advice.
- If you experience the sensation of you or the room spinning this is **vertigo,** and treatment is available, be specific when discussing your symptoms with your doctor.

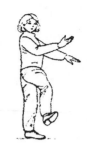

Solutions for Poor Balance

If your doctor agrees;

- Start with the beginner exercises found on page 41.

- Your exercise program should include strengthening exercises, balance exercises and walking.

- **Take a Tai Chi Class or balance exercise class.**

  ❖ Tai Chi is a form of balance exercises that emphases weight shifting while standing.

  ❖ No matter what your age studies indicate that Tai Chi may help to improve balance, and reduce the fear of falling.

- See page 39 on how to find and evaluate exercise classes.
- Join an evidence based fall prevention program (if available in your community) Call your local Area Agency on Aging. See appendix.

Solutions for Poor Balance

Don't multi-task: Doing two things at once affects balance, including walking and talking on cell phones.

Use a pill organizer (available at local pharmacies) to help keep track of time and dosage of medications. Mistakes with medications can interfere with balance and cause a fall.

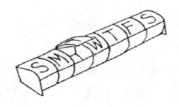

Limit alcohol. Check with your doctor. Check with your pharmacist for any drug/alcohol interaction; including over the counter medications.

If you are lightheaded when first standing up wait a minute before walking; this should give your body a chance to adjust. (The same holds true when first sitting up in bed.) This is a hot spot that needs to be discussed with your doctor.

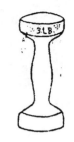

Strength

Found: The Fountain of Youth

Found: The Fountain of Youth

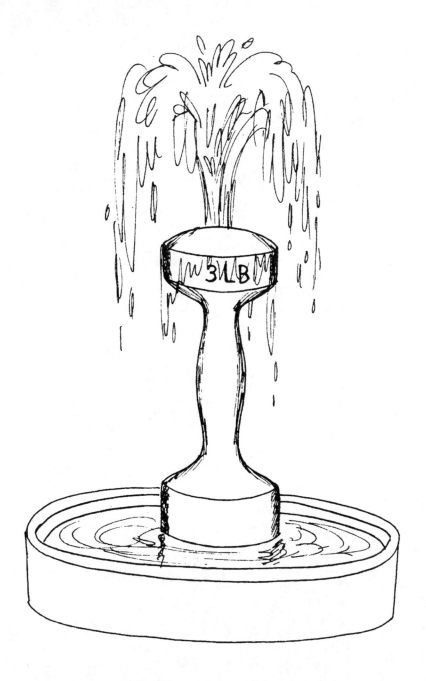

Strength

Do you/Are you???

- get proper nutrition
- drink enough fluids
- assume you are too old to exercise
- have muscle instead of fat
- think exercise must be intense to make a difference
- limber and not stiff
- lift weights
- walk daily
- able to stand up easily

Hot Spot
Loss of Strength

Muscle strength starts to decrease after age 40. Without exercise fat replaces muscle.

Hot spots are:
- poor nutrition and hydration
- difficulty getting out of a chair/middle seat of a sofa
- difficulty climbing a flight of stairs because leg muscles become tired
- walking hesitantly
- sedentary life style

Leg weakness is considered a fall risk factor.

Seventy-five year old Sylvia went to her doctor with complaints of not feeling like herself. Her daily gardening was becoming more of a chore instead of a pleasure. After evaluation it was determined that Sylvia was in good health but was losing muscle strength from lack of targeted exercise. Her doctor advised her to join a strengthening program at her local YMCA. After two months Sylvia's friends wanted to know her secret for her new youthful look.

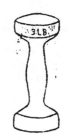

Solutions for Loss of Strength

Proper nutrition is essential for healthy aging and for providing the building blocks for strength.
- If you have an illness, difficulty swallowing or condition that limits the kind of food you eat then see your physician, he may recommend seeing a registered dietician.
- If you are having difficulty chewing because of your teeth see your dentist because oral health affects nutrition.

Adequate hydration is required for good health.
- As you age the need for fluid remains but the ability to feel thirst may decline.
- Fluids can include water, juice, soup, milk and other non-alcoholic beverages.

Strength training is one of the most effective and easy ways to decrease fall risk. Talk to your doctor about starting a strengthening program.

- Regardless of age, strength can be increased! The results occur very quickly—there will be a change in your strength, appearance, walking and motivation.
- Strength training is for all ages; we know 90 year olds who lift weights.
- Increasing strength in leg muscles enables us to continue to climb stairs and get out of chairs easily.
- Increasing strength reduces flabbiness, increases muscle tone and prevents bone loss.

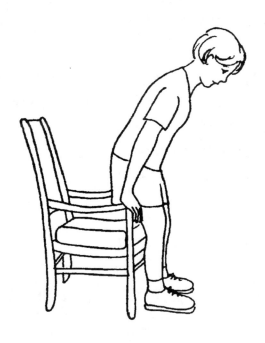

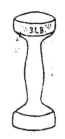

Solutions for Loss of Strength

**Strength training is for all ages!
Studies show that strength can be increased at any age!
Increasing strength can help reduce fall risk.**

Start walking! Walking combined with strength training insures that we keep moving.
- wear your walking shoes (good comfortable support)
- open the door and start today
- walk at a moderate pace

(see walking tips on page 53)

Stretching A mild stretching yoga class is a fun way to increase flexibility. Look for a class that emphasizes gentle stretching.

Begin exercising today...it is easier than you think!

- A book that will increase your motivation regardless of your age is, *Age-Defying Fitness: Making the Most of Your Body for the Rest of Your Life* by Marilyn Moffat PT, PhD and Carole B. Lewis PT, PhD.

- Start by turning to the exercise section that follows ---- remember these eight exercises are just to get you started.

- Places to inquire about exercise/strengthening/balance programs:
  Local Area Agency on Agency
  Senior Center
  Health/Fitness Club/YMCA
  High School Adult Education
  Hospital Wellness Center
  Friends/word of mouth
  Local Health Department

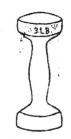

Solutions for Loss of Strength

Join a group exercise program.

- Ask to observe a class to determine if it is what you are looking for.
  - ❖ Evaluate the teaching style, class size and age of participates to see if it suits your needs.
  - ❖ Speak to the instructor and discuss your exercise background to determine if this class is what you want.
  - ❖ Health club statistics show one out of four members are over the age of 55.
  - ❖ Silver Sneakers is the name of a program geared to seniors being offered at some health clubs/YMCA. There may be a wide variation in what this class includes from club to club so you need to evaluate the class before joining.
  - ❖ The American College of Sports Medicine, ACSM, trains and certifies people to work with older adults. Ask the facility if it has someone certified to work with older adults.
- If you are home bound, there are DVDs, CDs and videos available to get you started.

Solutions for Loss of Strength

A physical therapist can establish an exercise program <u>specific to your needs</u>; this is especially beneficial if disease, medical conditions or physical limitations are present. In some states you will need a doctor's referral to be seen by a physical therapist but it is well worth the extra effort.

- To find a therapist call your local hospital's outpatient physical therapy department, look in the yellow pages, ask friends/doctor for recommendations, or visit the American Physical Therapy Association's web site (www.apta.org).

- Some physical therapists have specialty certification in geriatrics, orthopedics, cardiopulmonary, or neurology. Request a specialty for your needs.

- Ask to see a therapist who is experienced in your problem area or call the APTA 1 800 999-2782.

Exercise
Improve strength, balance and posture

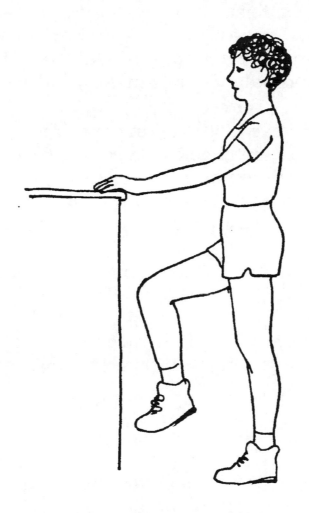

One – Two – Three …

The only equipment needed is you and your kitchen counter or sturdy chair.

<u>The following eight exercises are only to get you started</u>. They are beginning exercises targeted to improve your balance, strength and posture. You should progress at your own rate to an organized program that suits your needs and includes strength and balance training.

Before beginning any exercise/walking or joining an exercise/walking program check with your physician. If you have any medical condition or are not sure if you should perform certain exercises, discuss your concerns with your physician and/or physical therapist.

- Wear comfortable clothes and well fitting shoes that offer good support.

- Do these exercises at your kitchen counter or sturdy chair. Stop if you are dizzy, feel pain or are short of breath.

- Do these exercises 3 times a week.

- Put a check mark on your calendar when you exercise. It only takes 21 days to make a habit, so...

Let's Begin!

1. **Rocking Feet** - Stand facing kitchen counter/chair, feet shoulder width apart and hold on as needed.
   - keep knees soft (don't lock your knees)
   - rock forward onto the balls of your feet, raising your heels, hold for a count of three
   - keep standing straight, rock backwards onto your heels, lifting your toes, hold for count of three
   - repeat slowly 5-10 times

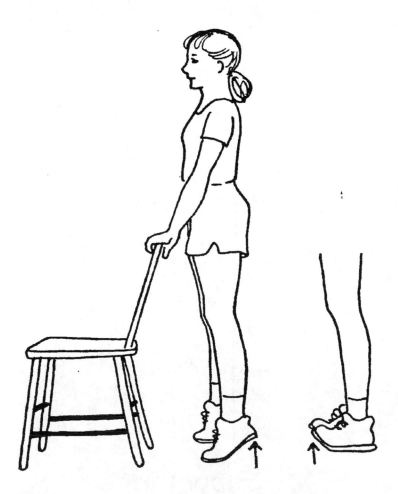

Rocking Feet

2. Slow March - Stand facing kitchen counter or chair with your feet about 6 inches apart and hold on with one or two hands as needed.

- keeping knees soft (don't lock knees)
- lift one knee up in a slow marching motion
- hold for a count of five as you balance on supporting leg
- slowly lower leg back to standing position
- pause
- repeat with other leg
- do 5-10 repetitions

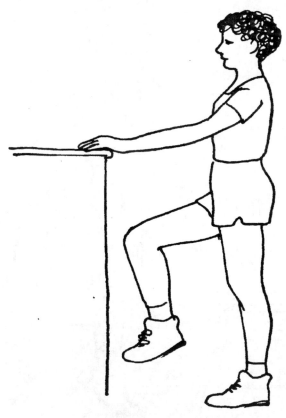

Slow march

3. Walking Backwards - Stand sideways by your kitchen counter and if needed rest your hand on counter.
- slowly walk backwards to the end of the counter
- pause, turn and repeat
- start by taking small steps and as you feel more comfortable increase to larger steps
- do 5-10 repetitions

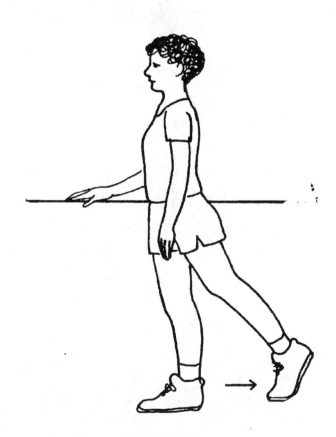

Walking Backwards

4. Heel-toe walking - Stand sideways next to kitchen counter or wall, hold on as needed.

- place one foot in front of the other so the heel of one shoe touches the toe of the other shoe (heel to toe pattern)
- walk forward looking straight ahead using a heel to toe pattern
- pause, turn, repeat
- do 10 to 20 steps, 2 to 3 repetitions

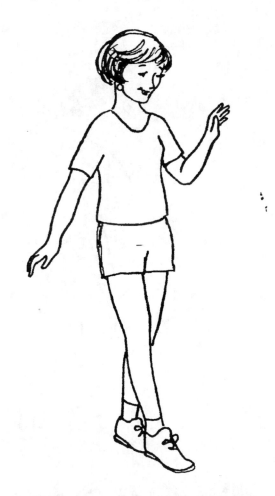

Heel Toe Walking

5. Walking Sideways - Stand facing kitchen counter with your feet and knees facing forward. Don't turn your feet out. Hold on with one or two hands as needed.

- while keeping your toes and knees pointing straight ahead walk sideways to the end of the counter, pause
- then walk sideways back to starting position, pause
- repeat 5-10 times in each direction

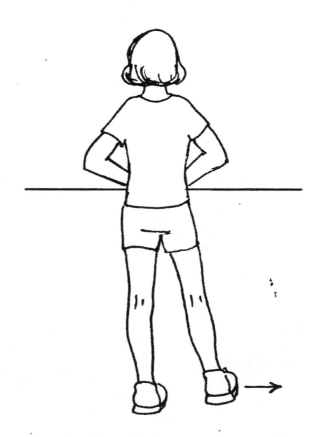

Walking Sideways

6. Sit to Stand-Stand to Sit

- sit in a straight back chair with your arms crossed over your chest
- lean forward slowly and straighten up to stand (the push comes from your legs)
- once standing bend forward at your waist and slowly lower yourself down to sit while keeping your arms crossed over your chest, do not flop down, control it, and don't hold your breath
- work up to 5 to 10 repetitions

If you are unable to do this with your arms crossed then use the armrests of the chair to help you stand, but your goal is to use your arms less and your legs more.

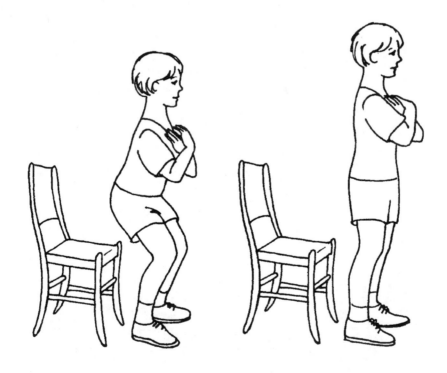

Sit to Stand - Stand to Sit

7. Chin Tuck
While sitting or standing.
- tuck your chin towards your chest and pull your head slightly back while squeezing shoulder blades together
- hold for five seconds and breathe
- repeat 5 to 10 times
- get in the habit of doing this both standing and sitting

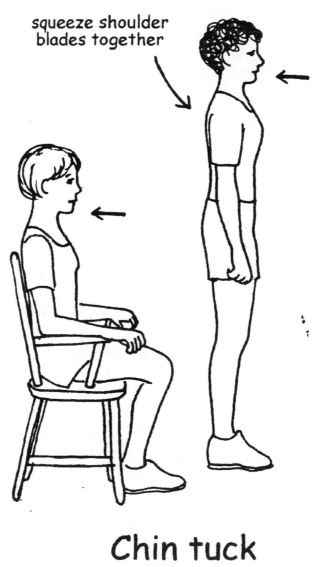

squeeze shoulder blades together

Chin tuck

8. Stair Climbing

- hold onto railing and step up onto stair with your left foot
- then bring right foot up onto same stair
- step back down off stair with your left foot
- then step down off stair with your right foot
- repeat 5-10 times with right leg leading and then 5-10 times with left leg leading

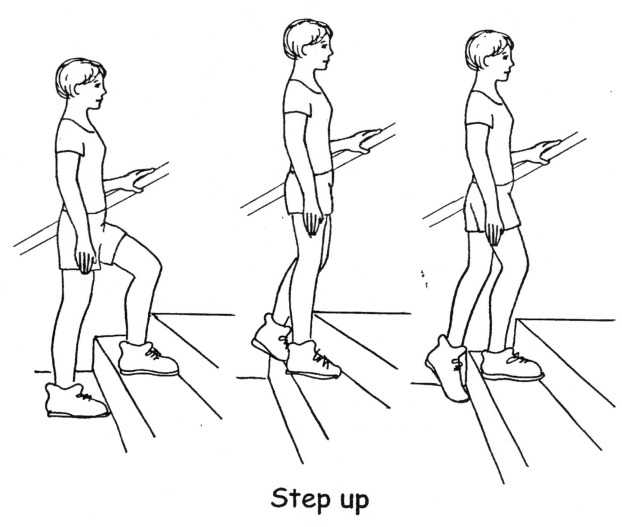

Step up

50

Exercise Review

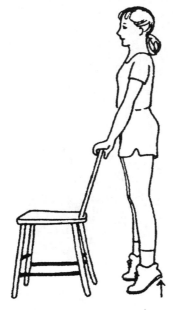

Rocking Feet

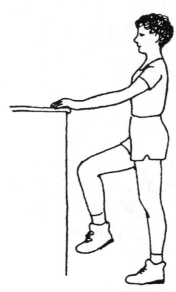

Slow march

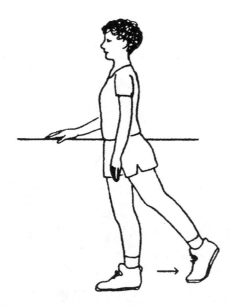

Walking Backwards

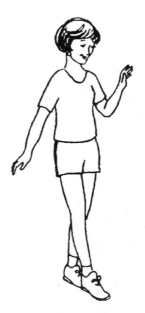

Heel Toe Walking

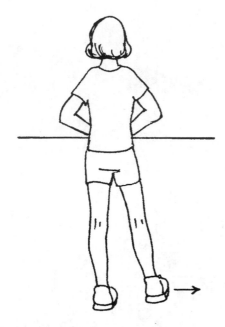

Walking Sideways

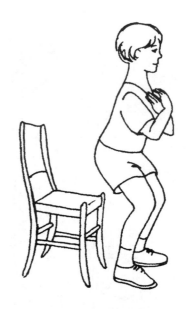

Sit to Stand

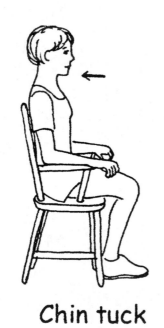

Chin tuck

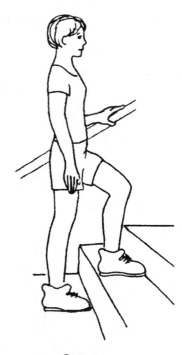

Step up

Walking For Exercise

Walking Tips

In addition to these exercises make walking part of your exercise routine. (first check with your doctor)

Wear a well fitting shoe/sneaker with good support (cross trainer or walking sneaker) that has...

- room for your toes to wiggle
- no slipping at heel
- arch of shoe matching your foot arch
- well cushioned insert
- bend at forefoot not midfoot
- laces/velcro so you can control fit
- sole that's not too 'grippy'

Open the door and start today ...

- start with 5-10 minutes
- walk at a moderate pace
- if you usually use a cane take it along (make sure it is the right size for you and you know how to properly use it, if needed see a PT)
- try to walk on sidewalks and level surfaces
- remember to stand straight, do your chin tuck while walking
- your goal is to make walking a daily habit

This is intended to keep you active not as a cardio-vascular exercise; however should you develop any discomfort, dizziness, joint pain, chest pain or shortness of breath then stop walking and consult with your doctor.

Questions?

1. What should I wear?
Comfortable clothes with pockets and supportive walking shoes. Some people use a fanny pack around their waist or carry a light weight tote bag.

2. What should I bring with me?
Carry ID, cell phone, money and tissues. Some people enjoy walking with a friend. Dogs usually take their owners for a walk.

3. Do I need a water bottle?
Yes, if you want, but since this is a beginning program with short walks you could drink a glass of water before you start out and another when you get home.

4. Should I stretch before walking?
It is not necessary at this level of beginning walking and we don't want to bog you down with so many things to do that you don't go for that walk.

5. Are there walking clubs?
Yes many communities have walking clubs. Check with your local mall, YMCA, or senior citizen center. These are especially useful on days you would not walk outdoors; when it is cold, windy, rainy or hot.

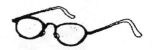

Vision

What Do You See?

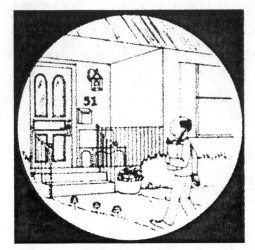

Cataracts

What Do You See?

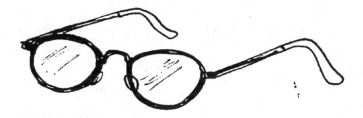

Glaucoma

Macular degeneration

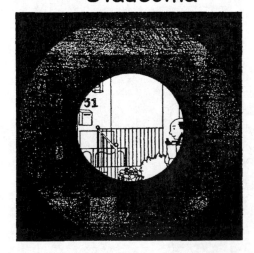

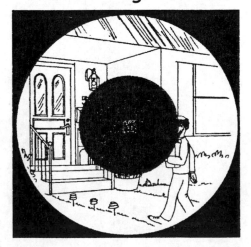

Vision

Do you/Are you???

- see an ophthalmologist/optometrist yearly
- wear glasses or have a new prescription
- have glasses that fit properly
- notice temporary blindness when entering a dark room
- have difficulty seeing at night
- have trouble with glare
- have difficulty with depth perception
- knowledgeable about common causes of blindness

Vision prevents us from tripping over obstacles and is also an important component of balance. It is more difficult to maintain balance with eyes closed than with them open. That is why we recommend having good lighting, cool burning night-lights, and flashlights throughout your home. (Night-lights without cool burning bulbs can be a fire hazard if they come in contact with materials.)

Hot Spot
Vision Changes

Macular degeneration is the leading cause of legal blindness.
Half of all Americans develop cataracts by age 80.
(The Vision Council of America)

Hot spots are
- vision changes
- new prescription glasses
- slow vision adaptation (adjusting to changes in levels of light)
- glare interfering with vision
- poor depth perception
- medical conditions/low vision
- adapting to new multifocal glasses on stairs

Not having vision checked/eye examines at least yearly is considered a fall risk factor.

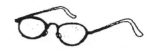

Solutions for Changes in Vision

Know who's who:
- An **ophthalmologist** is a physician who specializes in medical/surgical treatment of eye diseases.
- An **optometrist** (O.D.) does comprehensive eye and vision examinations, prescribes corrective lenses and can diagnose and treat vision disorders.
- An **optician** makes eyeglasses and fills ophthalmic prescriptions.

Have a yearly eye exam by your ophthalmologist or optometrist for any needed vision corrections and to check for common eye changes that could lead to low vision.
- If you notice any vision changes, see your vision specialist immediately

Symptoms to report to your eye doctor. Some are normal changes with aging but let your doctor diagnose.
- night blindness
- problem with depth perception (one example of depth perception is the ability to judge the height of steps)
- changes with peripheral vision (bumping into things)
- problem with visual contrast (one example of visual contrast is the ability to distinguish a curb from flat pavement)
- slowness of eyes adapting to darkness
- increased sensitivity to glare

If you wear glasses
- be careful when wearing a new prescription
- report any problems immediately, especially dizziness
- the new progressive/multifocal lenses have been readily received by many, however, some people have difficulty adjusting to these; practice wearing them in familiar surroundings
- progressive lenses and bifocals that don't fit can slip down your nose and cause distortions and missteps
- take care when on stairs, where you look through the lens can affect depth perception

Solutions for slow vision adaptation
- when entering a dark room or when entering the house from being outdoors on a sunny day give your eyes time to adjust to the different light level
- do not attempt to continue walking until your eyes have adapted to the change in light
- a helpful hint is to carry a small flashlight with you when you go to the movies, theater, etc.

Ways to reduce glare
- use blinds/sheer curtains
- use sconce lighting on walls
- have a matte floor finish
- wear sunglasses outdoors
- cover glass top tables with cloth runners

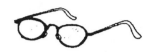

Solutions for Vision
Ways to enhance depth perception

- Highlight step edges, use contrasting colored tape. (Place a small piece on step edges, see illustration) Many falls occur on one and two step stairs.
- Request curbs and outside steps to be highlighted in your community and in rental properties.

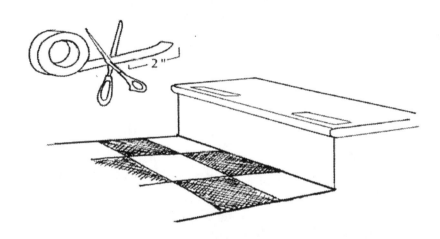

Be knowledgeable of conditions that affect vision

- Poor vision usually improves with corrective lenses.
- Low vision is a loss of vision that cannot be corrected with glasses. Resources are available – catalogs such as Independent Living, LightHouse and Maxiaids
- The most common causes of low vision are cataracts, macular degeneration, glaucoma and vision changes from diabetes.

Examples of visual conditions.

Cataracts

Cataracts can develop gradually and painlessly. Some symptoms of cataracts include:
- hazy, blurry, fuzzy vision
- difficulty seeing at night
- increased sensitivity to glare
- double vision
- lights appear to have halos around them
  illustration of vision affected by cataracts

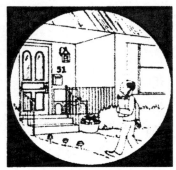

Cataracts

Diabetes –diabetic retinopathy

If you have diabetes, you know that the best way to prevent vision loss is by controlling your blood sugar levels.
- People with diabetes need to control their blood sugar and keep their blood pressure within normal ranges to prevent vision loss.
- Visit the ophthalmologist on a regular basis.

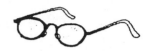

Glaucoma

- Glaucoma is a disorder in which the pressure in the eyeball increases and damages the optic nerve which causes a loss of vision.

- Glaucoma has no known cause, but it sometimes runs in families.

- Usually there are no early symptoms, but early detection can slow down progression of the disease.

- Later symptoms include a loss of peripheral vision, blind spots in the visual field, headaches or increasing difficulty adapting to darkness.

Illustration of vision with glaucoma

Glaucoma

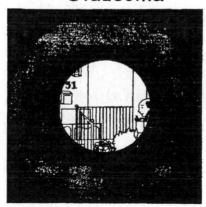

Macular Degeneration

Macular degeneration is a condition in which the macula (the central area of the retina) degenerates. This condition can slowly or suddenly cause a painless loss of central vision. Sometimes a symptom is straight lines appear wavy. Illustration of vision with macular degeneration.

Macular degeneration

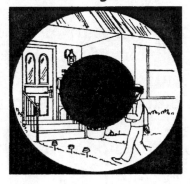

FYI Ears, vision and balance

Changes in hearing, ear aches, or dizziness should be evaluated by your doctor as these conditions may affect balance. The inner ear works together with the visual and proprioceptive systems to maintain balance.

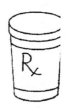

Medications/Alcohol

Know Their Effects

Know Their Effects

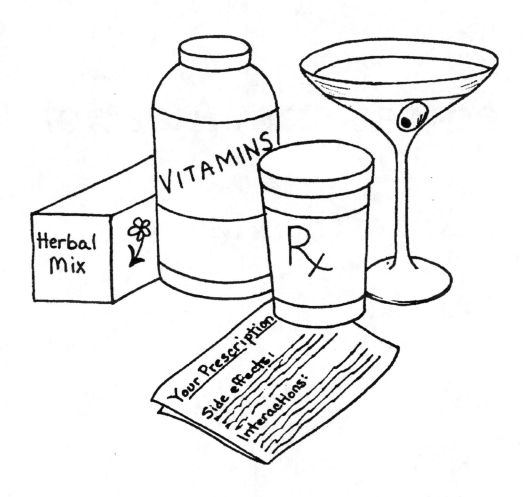

Medications/Alcohol

Do you???

- take three or more medications including over the counter (OTC) non-prescription medications
- take any sleeping medications, (prescription or OTC)
- comply with medication dose and frequency
- use a pill organizer
- keep a current list of medications in your wallet and in your home on your refrigerator (ask your pharmacist about vial of life medical information storage)
- keep all medications in their original container (except for those in your pill organizer)
- discard outdated medications
- keep your doctor informed of all the medications you take
- drink alcohol

Hot Spot
Medications/Alcohol

Hot Spots are:

- medications that slow reaction time (such as sleeping pills) the slower our reaction time the more difficult it becomes to "catch our balance"
- taking 3 or more medications on a daily basis is considered a fall risk factor
- not informing doctor about taking over the counter medications
- not following correct dosage and time schedule
- alcohol delays reaction time and always impairs balance and coordination
- alcohol and some medications interact badly

Taking three or more medications on a daily basis is considered a fall risk factor.

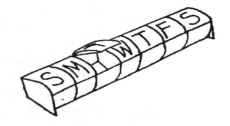

Solutions for Medications/Alcohol

There are over 150 frequently prescribed medications and over the counter medications. Misuse may affect balance and cause a fall. Take medications as prescribed!

Keep an updated list of all medications and dosages, both prescription and over the counter. **FYI** There are programs such as, "Vial of Life", which are designed to be placed on your refrigerator if there is a medical emergency.

Review medications and possible interactions with your doctor and pharmacist, including OTC medications.

Call your doctor if you find that you are **sluggish or dizzy** on your medications.

Use a **pill organizer** to keep track of time and dosage. Pill organizers are available at pharmacies and they come in many different styles.

Solutions for Medications/Alcohol

Use sleep medications with caution as they can interfere with your balance.
- maybe you will not need sleep medications if you limit daytime napping and caffeine consumption
- if tired during the day take a ten minute break for relaxation instead of a nap, or limit naps to ten minutes
- make sure to tell doctor about any OTC sleeping aids

If you consume alcohol, limit it to one drink a day.
Check with your pharmacist for any drug interaction.
- common drugs, both prescription and over the counter, such as antidepressants and sleeping medications interact badly with alcohol
- we can become tipsy with very little alcohol
- as we age our blood alcohol level takes longer to drop and return to normal
- alcohol delays reflexes and can turn a trip into a fall

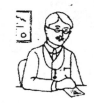

Doctor Relationship

Do You Tell Your Doctor Everything?

Do You Tell Your Doctor Everything?

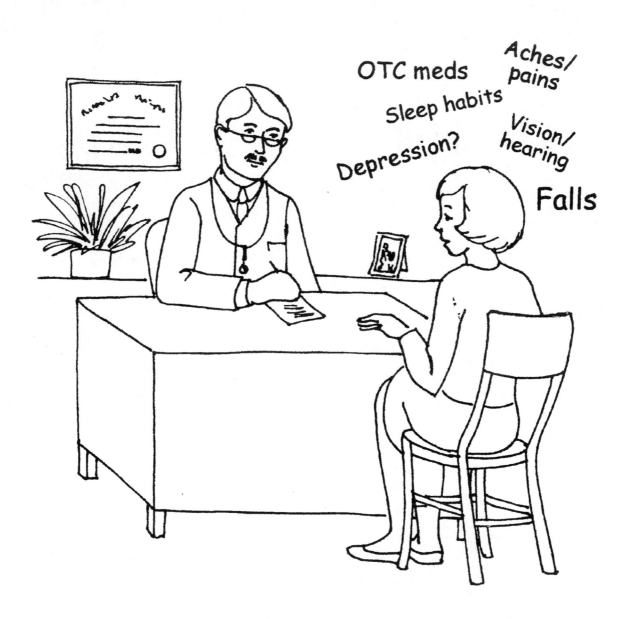

OTC meds

Aches/pains

Sleep habits

Depression?

Vision/hearing

Falls

Doctor Relationship

Do you/Are you???
- know how to select a doctor
- have a comfortable relationship with your doctor
- able to discuss all of your concerns
- discuss falls and fear of falling
- leave an office visit with a clear understanding of treatment and medications
- proactive in seeking medical care

Hot Spot
Poor Communication with Your Doctor

Hot spots are

- not feeling comfortable/confident with your doctor
- being told, "You are aging, what do you expect?"
- feeling dismissed
- not having your questions written down
- being hurried and unable to ask questions
- leaving your questions to the end of the exam
- not discussing all your concerns with your doctor
- not visiting your doctor for an examination after a fall including falls without any apparent injury

Haven fallen in the past six months is a fall risk factor.

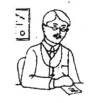

Solutions for Poor Communication with Doctor

Find a **doctor who addresses your concerns**.
- Ask your friends for recommendations.
- Call your local hospital or the American Medical Association for their 'find a doctor service'.
- Some doctors specialize in aging and are called geriatricians.

Have a **family member or friend accompany you** on doctor visits.
- This can lessen your anxiety and help create a more relaxed atmosphere.
- They can take notes for you to keep in your records and to review after your appointment.

Be proactive in maintaining your health.
- Your doctor is not a mind reader. He depends on you to tell him how you feel.
- Tell him what is on your mind; don't just wait for him to ask questions.
- Discuss financial concerns that might stop you from taking medication as prescribed.

Arrive prepared for your medical appointments with your **questions and concerns written down.** Such as...

- any falls, fear of falling or changes in balance
- urinary/bowel changes (urgency has been linked to falls, this can be treated)
- depression/changes in cognition/memory
- alcohol use
- vision/hearing changes
- sleeping habits
- dizziness/vertigo
- medications; prescription and over the counter
- do not wait until the end of the visit to discuss your concerns

Things to discuss about falls:

- pain or discomfort from a fall
- circumstances surrounding fall
- time of day fall occurred
- location-where you fell
- shoes/clothing worn when you fell
- activity engaged in at time of fall
- how you where feeling
- medications taken that day

Leave office visit with clear understanding and **written instructions** of treatment and/or medications.

- Date this and keep in your files.
- Ask for copies of any medical tests and keep in your personal records.
- Update medication list.

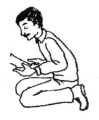

Shoes/Feet

Does the Shoe Fit?

Does the Shoe Fit?

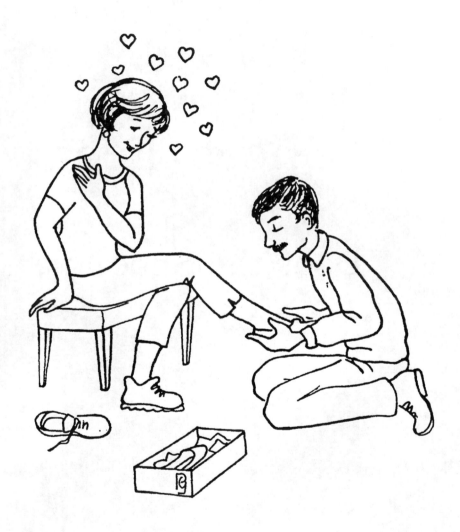

Shoes/Feet

Do you/Have you???

- pain free feet
- proper fitting shoes
- check the soles and heels of your shoes for wear
- trendy/dress shoes
- open back shoes
- foot problems; bunions, flat feet etc.

There are 26 bones and 30 joints that make up the foot and ankle. Your feet must have a well fitting shoe. Do not ignore or live with foot pain. (There are plenty of companies that specialize in making a comfortable, proper fitting shoe, brands such as; SAS, New Balance, Rockport and Naturalizer.)

Hot Spot
Poor Fitting Shoes

Poor fitting shoes can cause painful feet, poor balance, and could increase your risk of a fall.

Hot Spots are:
- painful feet
- poor fitting shoes
- worn out soles and heels of shoes
- slippery soles and heels of shoes
- smooth leather bottom shoes
- shoes with thick heavy soles
- high heels
- mules (shoes without backs)
- slippers
- flip-flops
- sandals, open toe and open back

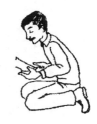

Solution for Shoes/Feet

Don't accept painful feet.
- If you have foot pain see your podiatrist.
- If you have arthritis in your feet see a rheumatologist.
- Discuss your personal foot care needs with your doctor/podiatrist.
- Don't ignore foot pain because it will affect your balance, posture and walking.
- Everyone with diabetes needs to be instructed in proper foot care and monitored by a doctor as diabetes can diminish sensation and circulation in your feet.
- For those of you who have diabetes it is crucial that your shoes fit properly.

Solutions for Shoes/Feet

Have a qualified person fit your shoes.

- patronize a store that has a knowledgeable sales clerk or pedorthist, (pedorthists are board certified fitters who are knowledgeable in the design, fit and modifications of shoes)
- ask your podiatrist and friends for recommendations for shoes, stores and fitter
- look at the bottom of your old shoes and show it to your fitter, it will reveal a lot about your walking pattern and what you need in a shoe

Get a good fit.

- if the shoe does not fit at the store it will not fit later
- your shoes affect your ability to walk, how you walk, your balance, posture and comfort

What makes for a good fit?

- have your feet measured every time you buy shoes
- feet swell so the best fit is obtained in the afternoon
- get measured standing with full weight on both feet
- measure both feet, most of us have one foot larger than the other, fit for the larger foot and adjust the other shoe with a tongue or heel pad
- allow ¼ - ½ inch from the end of the shoe to the tip your longest toe
- the toe box needs to be wide enough so your toes do not overlap, and the heel should be snug in the shoe

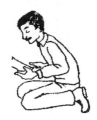

Solution for Shoes/Feet

Check out the soles and heels of your shoes.

- Look for a shoe with a **non-skid or rubber sole** but not too 'grippy', heavy or thick.
- Sometimes a crepe or **thick rubber sole is too 'grippy'** and can catch as you walk causing a trip.
- Some soles become slippery and smooth and are a fall hazard. Discard them.
- Some newer materials used in the heels can be very slippery so take notice of the heel as well as the sole and if it is slippery do not buy it.
- Men/women with smooth leather bottom shoes should sandpaper the soles or rub them against a sidewalk before wearing them.

High Heels

- Wearing shoes with a lower heel improves balance, but <u>do not quickly</u> switch from long time use of a shoe with a high heel to a flat shoe. You may experience a change in balance or calf pain due to stretching a shortened Achilles tendon. In fact, if you have never worn a flat shoe you will probably do better in a shoe with a small heel.

Solutions for Shoes/Feet

Slippers
- Wear well fitting slippers that have a rubber sole and a back, not sloppy fitting scuffs.
- Do not walk around the house with only stockings or socks on your feet, this is slippery and dangerous.

Sandals/Flip-Flops
- If you wear open toe sandals make sure they fit properly and have a flexible sole. However-
- The American Physical Therapy Association's (APTA) advices not to wear open-toed sandals as they can cause you to trip.(The sandal can catch at the toe and can cause a trip.)
- Flips-flops are fashionable but do not provide proper foot support, and can be slippery when wet (your foot can slip inside the flip flop causing a loss of balance).

Special circumstances If you have one leg shorter than the other a shoe lift can even out the discrepancy and will improve balance and walking. (See your orthopedist.)
- Orthotics (custom shoe inserts) are available to correct other foot problems and also improve balance and walking, see your podiatrist or physical therapist.

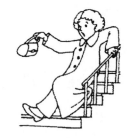

Clothing

Watch those Hemlines!

Watch Those Hemlines!

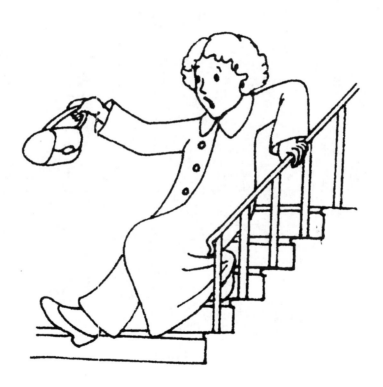

Clothing

Do you wear???

- ankle length dresses or skirts
- long coats
- long flowing robes
- wide leg pants
- flowing sleeves

**Hot Spot
Clothing**

Osteoporosis can produce a gradual loss in height.

One of our friends reported a near fall when descending the stairs of her church. Her heel caught the hem of her long coat. She was able to gracefully sit down instead of falling because she was holding the hand railing. Be careful when wearing long clothing on stairs, both going up and coming down.

Hot spots are:
- hemlines that are too long
- robes that are longer than mid-calf
- wide leg pants
- flowing sleeves
- not picking up a long skirt/coat on curbs and stairs

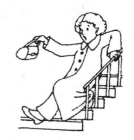

Solutions for Clothing

To avoid tripping on your clothes, check your hemlines each season. Not only is this fashionable but more importantly we can shrink with age and long hemlines are a tripping hazard.

While checking hemlines also check the length of your sleeves. Wide sleeves are not only a fire hazard when cooking; they also can cause a fall when they get caught on door handles and railings.

If you wear wide leg pants descend stairs carefully to avoid catching your foot in the excess material.

When wearing a long skirt or coat, lift it up when going up and down stairs and curbs to avoid stepping on it and falling.

Helpful Hints

Sit in a sturdy chair when dressing, not on the edge of the bed. The chair offers more support and you won't slip off the edge.

When standing don't bend over to tie your shoes or put on your stockings or socks. Sit down. A handy device is a long handle shoe horn. They are available at pharmacies and other surgical supply stores.

If you have difficulties managing your clothing and dressing independently consult an occupational therapist who can offer techniques and suggestions for safe and independent dressing. An occupational therapist is a professional who helps individuals achieve independence in activities of daily living. (See appendix.)

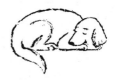

Pets

Are They Underfoot?

Are They Under Foot?

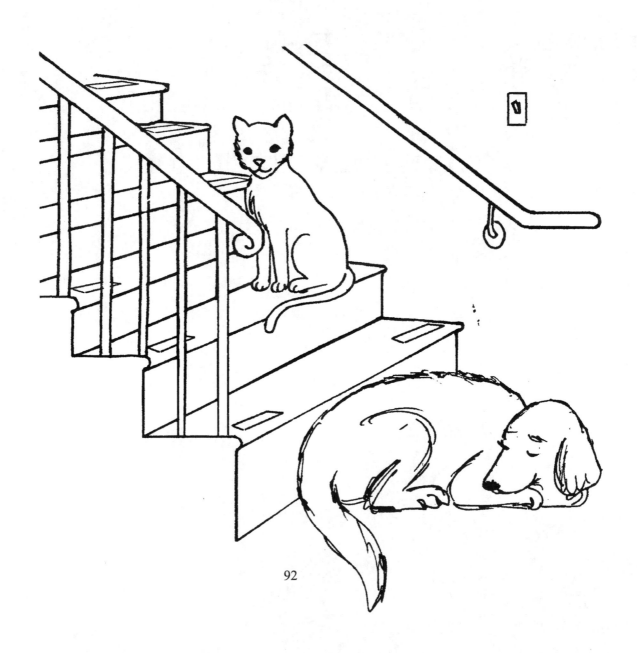

Pets

Do you have???

- an energetic puppy
- a sedentary dog
- a cat
- a zoo of a house

Hot Spot
Pets

Hot spots are:

- jumping Fido
- small animals under foot
- cats nestled on stairs
- a dog who walks you

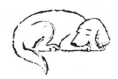

Solutions for Pets

Dog training can solve many dog and puppy problems.
- Don't let the dog train you; the dog wants you to train him.
- There are classes and videos/DVDs available; check with your local pet store.
- Training your dog is a lot of fun for both for the owner and the dog.
- A trained dog is a joy for life. An extra perk is both you and your dog will get your walking exercise.

If walking your dog is a problem, **enlist the help of dog walker.**
- Call your local pet store or veterinarian for names.
- If this is not an option then look into **fencing part of your yard**. There is standard fencing and invisible fencing available, check with your pet store for companies that provide this service.
- Use a chain that can be anchored to the ground that gives the dog freedom to roam and yet is confined to the yard.

Do not allow your cat or dog to sleep on the stairs, this is a tripping hazard.

Place collars with bells on your pets. This can alert you to their presence and prevent you from tripping on them.

Provide your veterinarian with information about who will care for your pet if you become ill.

Placing the litter box on top of a sturdy box will decrease the amount you have to bend. Make sure that your cat can still get to it.

There are many **helpful animal gadgets** available from your pet store and catalogs. Check them out. If bending is difficult there are elevated food bowls, timed release food bowls, etc. Many things that you never knew you needed.

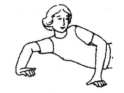

What To Do If You Fall

Take Inventory

What to do if you fall.

This is a review of what you read in the section on fear of falling. As we know not all falls can be prevented so we need to be prepared in what to do if we fall.

Look at illustrations on next page.

1. Don't panic. Take a deep breath and take inventory, make sure you are not injured. If you are not injured roll onto your side. If you are injured use your fall pendant or your reachable phone and call for assistance.

2. Get on to hands and knees.

3. Crawl, scoot, move along floor to a sturdy chair or couch (a low piece of furniture will provide the best support). If chair seat is too high you can always place hands under the cushions.

4. Place one foot flat on floor and curl the toes on the other foot so they are gripping the floor. Using your arms and legs to push up and stand.

5. Turn around and sit on the chair or couch.

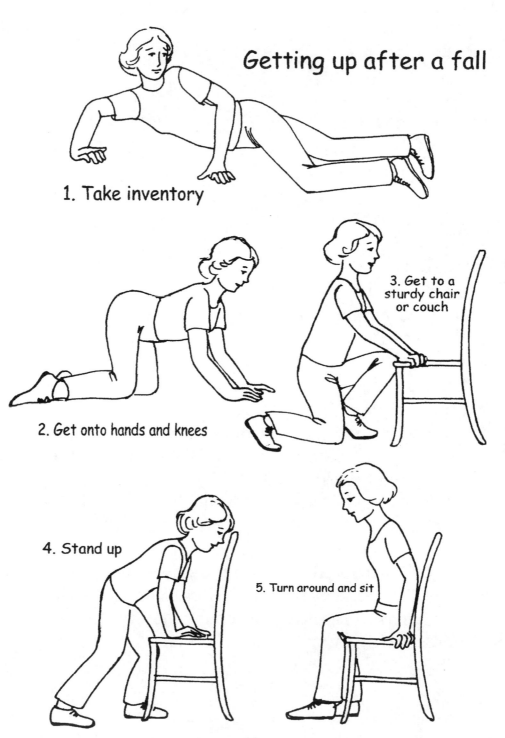

Getting up after a fall

1. Take inventory

2. Get onto hands and knees

3. Get to a sturdy chair or couch

4. Stand up

5. Turn around and sit

What to do if you are unable to get up:

- there is no rush
- take a deep breath
- determine what hurts
- use your accessible phone
- if you are using a fall pendant, then push the button and help will come

Fall Pendants:
- provide security
- can be worn as wrist watch, necklace, or clips on the belt, they should be water proof and worn in shower
- when activated it notifies a response center who then contacts a pre-designated doctor, family member or friend
- some companies that supply pendants include:
    American Medical Alarms 1 800 542-0438
    Life Alert 1 800 815-592
    Medical Alert Alarm System 1 800 906-0872
    Philips Lifeline 1 800 380-3111

Also, contact your local Area Agency on Aging, Red Cross or local Senior Citizen Center as they can often provide information on availability and cost of fall pendants. Sometimes renting is an option.

Evidence Based Fall Prevention Programs

There are many evidence based fall prevention programs throughout the country. To find if one is available in your area call your local senior center or area agency on aging.

Some of the program titles are:

Matter of Balance
Sure Steps
Don't Fall For IT
Stepping On
Step by Step
Stand Up and be Strong
Free from Falls
Fall Proof
HEROS
InSTEP

This list is not all inclusive and not all of these programs are available in all areas. If these particular fall prevention programs are not offered where you live most senior centers do offer exercise and balance programs such as Tai Chi.

Go to *www.n4a.org* for information on your local area agency on aging.

Congratulations!

You are now aware of your fall hot spots and when to seek medical attention. You have made your medical appointments, obtained your doctors approval to exercise, and called your local area agency on aging and senior centers for information on local fall prevention programs. That's a good start.

In addition you need to examine and correct your household environment. A comprehensive fall prevention/risk reduction program covers your home, body and life.

Review the following home safety checklist to identify and modify your household tripping hazards. Use the checklist to make your home safer and schedule needed repairs and improvements.

Home Safety Checklist

Entrance: Do you have.....
1. clear and level walkways?
2. secure and highlighted outdoor steps?
3. secure hand railings on both sides of steps?
4. easily managed door knobs, locks, and storm doors?
6. adequate lighting and motion detector lighting ?
7. an easily accessible mailbox?

Bathroom: Do you have.....
8. grab bars by the toilet and bath/shower area?
9. anti-slip surface or rubber mat on shower/bath floor?
10. a secure toilet seat at a comfortable height?
11. night-lights with a cool burning bulb?
10. an reachable phone?

Kitchen: Do you have....
13. frequently used items stored within your range of reach?
14. a non-slip mat by the sink?
15. a fire extinguisher that you know how to use?

Bedroom: Do you have.....

16. a bed that allows feet to touch the floor when sitting?
17. non-slip linens?
18. cool burning night-lights?
19. a clear path to the bathroom?
20. a flashlight on bedside table with extra fresh batteries?

Basement: Do you have...

21. a latched basement door?(guests may assume they are going outdoors and instead end up falling down basement stairs.)
22. well lit uncluttered stairs in good repair?
23. highlighted stairs with secure railings on both sides?
24. your washer and dryer in the most convenient location? It may be safer to relocate your washer and dryer upstairs.
25. an accessible phone reachable from the floor?

Furniture: Do you have...

26. sturdy tables? (no easily tipped-over pedestal tables)
27. coffee tables that are not too low to be a tripping hazard?
28. glass tabletops covered with a runner to reduce glare?
29. furniture that fits your body?

Stairs: Do you have...

30. hand railings that run the full length?
31. secure hand railings on both sides of stairs?
32. highlighted steps?

example apply a small piece of tape or spray paint the edge
of the step with a white or contrasting paint

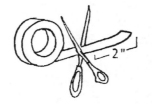

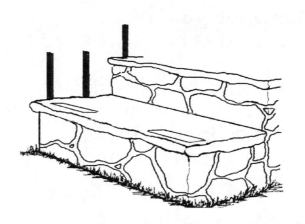

33. well lit stairs?
34. a light switch at the top and bottom of stairway?
35. uncluttered stairs, no stored items on steps?

Floors: Do you have....

36. beveled thresholds or highlighted thresholds?
37. slip resistant floors?
38. slip resistant area rugs?
39. carpets in good repair, not frayed or buckled?
40. glare free floors?
41. electrical cords out of walkways and not under rugs?

Lighting: Do you have....
42. light switches at all room entrances?
43. even-lighting in all rooms?
44. use bulbs with the highest recommended wattage?
45. night-lights in all bathrooms, bedrooms and hallways?
46. night-lights that use a cool burning bulb?
47. a flashlight on all levels of your home?
48. a power failure safety light?

Telephone: Do you have...
49. a phone that can be reached from the floor in every room?
50. at least one cordless phone?
51. at least one landline/corded phone?
52. an answering machine?
53. a list of emergency numbers by your phone and programmed into cell phone?

Garage/Car: Do you have...
54. stairs in good repair with highlighted steps and railings?
55. adequate lighting and uncluttered slip resistant floors?
56. automatic garage doors with emergency reverse?
57. a safe method to get in and out of your car?-take your time especially when the ground is uneven/slippery

Deck/Garden: Do you have.....
58. good body mechanics when you garden?
59. deck stairs highlighted?
60. secure railings by your deck stairs?

Home Emergencies: Do you know...

61. how to turn off the main water supply?
62. where your circuit breaker is?
63. a fire escape plan?
64. if your smoke alarm/carbon monoxide detector works?
65. where to place a water alarm?
66. if your battery operated radio and flashlight work?
67. to place emergency phone numbers next to phone?
68. an accessible fire extinguisher and know how to use it?

Home repairs: Do you have...

69. a contractor who is familiar with universal design? (Universal design refers to creating rooms, homes and products that can be used by everyone regardless of age, size, or physical ability. If you are planning to remodel, AARP has a free booklet upon request on universal design.)
70. a plan and timeline for home repairs and improvements?

Start today. Make your home repair notebook: Projects for today, this week, this month and this year.

For details on home safety tips see *Fall Prevention: Don't Let Your House Kick You Out!* ISBN 0-7414-3113-0

Catalogs

We do not endorse any of the following products or catalogs. We are including them for the reader to investigate and decide what fits their individual needs. Products, phone numbers and websites do change but to the best of our knowledge were accurate at the time of writing.

Abledata, www.abledata.com 1 800 227-0216 National database of assistive devices and rehabilitation equipment.

AliMed www.alimed.com 1 800 225-2610 The Help At Home catalog has health care products.

Bathroom systems: There are many companies that provide modular shower units and walk in baths. You can speak to your plumber and get materials from such companies as:

    Best Bath Systems- www.bestbath..com 1 800 727-9907
    Home Living Solutions www.homelivingsolutions.com 1 800 320-8182
    Independent Living USA www.independentlivingusa.com 1 800 403-7409
    Premier Baths www.premier-bathrooms.com 1 800 578-2899
    Safety Tubs www.safetytubs.com 1 877 304 2800

Bruce Medical Supply www.brucemedical.com 1 800 225-8446 Among many other items they carry the small "grab-it" grab bar and "auto touch lamps".

Diadot Disability Solutions www.diadot.com 973 875-5669 Provides grab bars in addition to many other home adaptive assistive equipment. They offer grab bars in many colors and in addition will install (they are located in northern New Jersey).

Fall Alert Devices
   American Medical Alarms 1 800 542-0438
   Medical Alert Alarm System 1 800 906 0872
   Life Alert 1800 815-5922
   Philips Lifeline 1 800 380-3111

FirstStreet for Boomers and Beyond www.firststreetonline.com 1800 704-1209
Catalog of useful products.

Independent Living Aids Inc, www.independentlivingaids.com 1800 537-2118 The
catalog offers magnifiers, lamps, and range of communication products.

Jeffers Pet Catalog, www.jefferspet.com 1800 533-3377

MaxiAids Catalog, www.maxiaids.com 1 800 522-6294 Offers adaptive products
designed for visually, hearing and physically impaired

Miles Kimball, www.mileskimball.com 1800 546-2255 Useful gadgets.

Walking Cane Company www.walkingcanepeople.com 1 888 399-4870 Presents
stylish canes and available accessories.

Sears Health and Wellness Catalog, www.searshealthandwellness.com 1800 326-
1750 Aids for living. Call for catalog.

Silvert's www.silverts.com 1 800 387-7088 The Easy-Wear, Easy-Care Clothing
Company. Clothing for easy dressing and special needs.

###

Resources

AARP (AARP), www.aarp.org 1-888 687-2277. A useful contact for information on aging successfully.

Administration On Aging, www.aoa.gov 1 202 619-0724. To find your local service call 1 800 677-1116 or check your phone book for the local **Division On Aging.** The local division can provide information on many topics including home repair programs, tax rebates, fall pendants, support groups and aging in place programs.

Age-Defying Fitness; Making the Most of Your Body for the Rest of Your Life
Marilyn Moffat, PT, PhD, FAPTA, Carole B. Lewis, PT, PhD, FAPTA, 2006.

AgingDeliberately www.agingdeliberately.com 1 206 780-8085. Liz Taylor, former Seattle Times columnist, now has her own informative website on aging deliberately.

American Diabetes Association, www.diabetes.org 1 800 342-2383.

American Geriatric Society, www.americangeriatrics.org 1 212 308-1414. Their mission is to improve the health, independence and quality of life of all older people.

American Medical Association, www.ama-assn.org 1 800 621-8335. They have a link to help find a doctor.

American Occupational Therapy Association (AOTA), www.aota.org 301 652-2682 or 1 800 377-8555. Can help locate an occupational therapist, OT, in your area.

American Physical Therapy Association (APTA), www.apta.org 1 800 999-2782. Can help locate a physical therapist, PT, in your area.

American Society on Aging, www.asaging.org 1 800 537-9728. Offers information and links on aging.

American Speech-Language-Hearing Association (ASHA), www.asha.org 1 800 638-8255. They will provide material on hearing and balance and links for products.

Brain Injury Association of New Jersey, www.bianj.org 1 800 669-4323 Provides fall prevention information to the community through "Heads Up! Seniors".

Centers for Disease Control and Prevention, National Center for Injury Prevention and Control **http://www.cdc.gov/ncipc/duip/preventadultfalls.htm** Provides information, fact sheets and brochures about falls.

Children of Aging Parents, www.caps4caregivers.org 1 800 227-7294. A national nonprofit whose mission is to assist caregivers with information on healthcare.

Fall Prevention Center of Excellence, www.stopfalls.org 1 213 740-1364. Their mission is to identify best practices in fall prevention and to help communities offer fall prevention programs to older people who are at risk of falling.
Fall Proof: A Comprehensive Balance and Mobility Training Program, Debra J. Rose 2003.

FOLO Families of Loved Ones, www.familiesoflovedones.com Quarterly magazine devoted to strategies and resources for caregivers. Publisher Cantwell Media LLC.

Home Safety Council, www.homesafetycouncil.org 1 888 245-1527. This site deals with home safety concerns. Their mission is to educate people of all ages to be safe in and around their homes.

Lighthouse, Vision Connection, www.lighthouse.org 1800 829-0500. Provides information about low vision and further vision links.

Mayo Clinic, www.mayoclinic.com Website only. Has information on many topics including osteoporosis and exercise.

National Arthritis Foundation, www.arthritis.org 1 800-283-7800

National Association of Professional Geriatric Care Managers, www.caremanager.org 1 520 881-8008. This organization can help locate a geriatric care manger in your area. A geriatric care manager organizes and oversees needed care giving services.

National Council on Aging, www.ncoa.org 1202 479-1200. Serves as a contact organization to improve seniors' lives. The National Council on Aging, Center for Healthy Aging developed Falls Free Coalition. The Falls Free Coalition is a group of national organizations and state coalitions working to reduce the growing number of falls and fall-related injuries among older adults.

National Family Caregivers Association, www.thefamilycaregiver.org 1 800 896-3650. Helpful site for those caring for an older or disabled relative.

National Institute of Health/National Institute On Aging, www.nih.gov/nia 1 800 222-2225. Provides information on health and aging. You can request their free booklet: *Exercise: A Guide from the National Institute on Aging.*

National Institutes of Health, Osteoporosis and Related Bone Disease, www.osteo.org 1-800 624-2663. Will send a free copy of a booklet on bone health.

National Parkinson Foundation, www.parkinson.org 1 800 327-4545 Will provide free booklets on dealing with Parkinson's disease.

National Resource Center for Safe Aging, (NRCSA), www.safeaging.org 1 619 594-0986. Increases awareness about injuries among older Americans.

National Resource Center on Supportive Housing and Home Modifications, www.homemods.org 1 213 740-1364. Provides housing modification information and pertinent links.

Osteoporosis, An Exercise Guide, Margie Bessiginger, MS, PT 1998.

Strong Women Stay Young, Miriam E. Nelson, PhD 2000.

Strong Women, Strong Bones, Miriam E. Nelson PhD, Everything you need to know to prevent, treat and beat osteoporosis. 2000.

Walk Tall, An Exercise Program for the Prevention, and Treatment of Osteoporosis, **Sara Meeks,** PT, GCS 1999.

References

American Geriatrics Society Panel on Fall Prevention, Guideline for the Prevention of Falls in Older Persons. *Journal of the American Geriatrics Society* 49:664-672, 2001.

Centers for Disease Control and Prevention. Falls Among older Adults: An Overview. Available at http://www.cdc.gov./ncipc/factsheets/adultsfalls.htm.

CDC *Preventing Falls: How to Develop Community-based Fall Prevention Programs for Older Adults.* 2008.

CDC *Preventing Falls: What Works: A CDC Compendium of Effective Community-based Interventions from Around the World.* 2008.

Day L, Fildes B, Gordon I, Fitzharris M, Flamer M, Lord S. Randomized factorial trial of falls prevention among older people living in their own homes. *British Medical Journal.* 2002 Jul 20;325(7356):128-33.
    Authors' conclusion: Group based exercise was the most effective single intervention tested. Falls were also reduced by the addition of home hazard management and vision management.

Fall Prevention Center of Excellence. Fall Prevention Intensive: Senior Injury Prevention Conference. May 9, 2007. Laurence Z. Rubenstein, MD, MPH Debra J. Rose, PhD Anna Quyen, Do Nguyen, OTD, OTR/L.

Fiatrone MA, O'Neill EF, Doyle Ryan, Clements KS, Solares GR, Nelson ME, et al. Exercise training and nutritional supplementations for physical frailty in very elderly people. *New England Journal of Medicine.* 1994;330(25):1769-75.
    Authors' conclusion: High-intensity resistance exercise training is an effective means of counteracting muscle weakness and physical frailty in elderly people.

Donat H, Ozcan A. Comparison of the effectiveness of two programs on older adults at risk of falling: unsupervised home exercise and supervised group exercise. *Clinical Rehabilitation.* 2007;21(3):273-283.

Authors' conclusions: In both the supervised exercise group and the unsupervised home exercise group, balance, functional mobility, and flexibility all improved among the subjects with risk of falling. Strength and proprioception, improved only within the supervised exercise group. Due to the ease of participation and the economical advantages, the authors suggest that unsupervised home exercises may be preferable to supervised exercise groups. In addition, the unsupervised home exercises can be enhanced by improving the strengthening and proprioceptive exercises.

Gillaspie LD, Gillespie WJ, Robertson MC, Lamb SE, Cumming RG, Rowe BH. Interventions for Preventing Falls in Elderly People. *The Cochrane Database of Systematic Reviews.* 1997, Issue 4. Art. No.: CD000340.

Summary: Interventions to prevent falls in elderly people can be effective. Multidisciplinary interventions targeting multiple risk factors are effective in reducing the incidence of falls, as is muscle strengthening combined with balance retraining, individually prescribed at home by a trained health professional. Tai Chi may also be effective. Home hazard assessment and modification by a health professional may reduce falls, especially in those with a history of falling. Cardiac pacing for fallers with cardio inhibitory carotid sinus hypersensitivity is likely to be beneficial, as is withdrawal of psychotropic medication. Individually tailored interventions delivered by a health professional are more effective than standard or group delivered programs.

Guccione, Andrew A., ed. *Geriatric Physical Therapy.* MO: Mosby, 2000.

Kannus P, Parkkari J, Niem S, Pasanen M, Palvanen M, Jarvinen M, et al. Prevention of hip fractures in elderly people with use of a hip protector. *New England Journal of Medicine.* 2000;343(21):1506-13.

Authors' conclusion: The risk of hip fracture can be reduced in frail elderly adults by the use of an anatomically designed external hip protector.

Koepsell TD, Wolf ME, Buchner DM, Kukull WA, LaCroix AZ, Tencer AF, Frankenfeld CL, Tautvydas M, Larson EB. Footwear Style and Risk of Falls in Older Adult. *Journal of the American Geriatrics Society.* 2004 Sep;52(9):1495-501.

   Authors Conclusion: Contrary to findings from gait-laboratory studies, athletic shoes were associated with relatively low risk of a fall in older adults during everyday activities. Fall risk was markedly increased when participants were not wearing shoes.

Leipzig RM, Cumming RG, Tinetti ME. Drugs and falls in older people: A systematic review and metaanalysis: I. Psychotropic drugs. *Journal of the American Geriatrics Society.* 1999;Jan:47(1):30-39.

   Authors' conclusion: There is a small, but consistent, association between the use of most classes of psychotropic drugs and falls.

Leipzig RM, Cumming RG, Tinetti ME. Drugs and falls in older people: A systematic review and metaanalysis: II. Cardiac and analgesic drugs. *Journal of the American Geriatrics..* 1999; Jan:47(1)40-50.

   Authors' conclusion: Older adults taking more than three or four medications were at increased risk of recurrent falls. As a result of the incidence of falls and their consequences in this population, programs designed to decrease medication use should be evaluated for their impact on fall rates.

Lord S, Dayhew J, Howland A. Multifocal Glasses Impair Edge-Contrast Sensitivity and Depth Perception and Increase the Risk of Falls in Older People. *Journal of the American Geriatrics Society.* 50 (11), 1760-1766.

   Authors' conclusion: The study findings indicate that multifocal glasses impair depth perception and edge-contrast sensitivity at critical distances for detecting obstacles in the environment. Older people may benefit from wearing nonmultifocal glasses when negotiating stairs and in unfamiliar settings outside the home.

Meeks PT, Sara. *Walk Tall! An Exercise Program for the Prevention and Treatment of Osteoporosis.* Florida: Triad, 1999.

Nelson PhD, Miriam. Strong *Women Stay Young.* New York: Bantam, 2000.

Nelson PhD, Miriam, Strong *Women Strong Bones.* New York: Bantam, 2000.

Notelovitz MD PhD, Morris. *Stand Tall! Every Women's Guide to Preventing and Treating Osteoporosis*. Florida: Triad, 1998.

Shumway-Cook A, Baldwin M, Polissar NL, Gruber W. Predicting the probability for falls in community dwelling older adults. *Phys Ther*. 1997; 77:812-819.
    Authors' conclusion: Assessing fall risk would allow identification of individuals who would likely benefit from services designed to reduce the risk for further injurious falls.

Tinetti ME, et al. Effect of dissemination of evidence in reducing injuries from falls. *New England Journal of Medicine*. 2008; 359: 252-61.
    Authors' conclusion: Dissemination of evidence about fall prevention, coupled with interventions to change clinical practice, may reduce fall-related injuries.

Tinetti ME, Speechley M.. Prevention of Falls Among the Elderly. *New England Journal of Medicine*. 1989;320(16):1055-9.
    Authors' conclusion: Most falls are neither random, unpredictable accidents nor the inevitable accompaniments of aging. The identification of elderly patients at risk for falling and intervention to minimize risk without compromising functional independence should receive a high priority in the health care of elderly persons.

Tinetti ME, Speechley M, Ginter SF. Risk Factors for Falls among Elderly Persons living in the community. *New England Journal of Medicine*. 1988;319(26):1701.
    Authors' conclusion: Multiple intrinsic, activity-related, and environmental factors were mentioned as contributing to most falls, thus calling into question the usefulness of simple categorization.

Tinetti ME, Baker DI, McAvay G, Claus EB, Garrett P, Gottschalk M, et al. A Multifactorial Intervention to Reduce the Risk of Falling among Elderly People living in the Community. *New England Journal of Medicine*. 1994; 331:821-7.
    Authors' conclusion: The multiple-risk-factor intervention strategy resulted in a significant reduction in the risk of falling among elderly persons in the community. In addition, the proportion of persons who had the targeted risk factors for falling was reduced in the intervention group, as compared with the control group. Thus, risk-factor modification may partially explain the reduction in the risk of falling. Risk factor reduction at least partially explained the decrease in the occurrence of falls.

Tinetti ME, Williams C. Falls, Injuries Due to Falls and the Risk of Admission to a Nursing Home. *New England Journal of Medicine.* 337(18):1279-84,1997 Oct.30.

 Authors' conclusion: Among older people living in the community falls are a strong predictor of placement in a skilled-nursing facility; interventions that prevent falls and their sequelae may therefore delay or reduce the frequency of nursing home admissions.

Wolf SL, Barnhart HX, Kutner NG, McNelly E, Coogler C, Xu T. Reducing frailty and falls in older persons: An investigation of Tai Chi and computerized balance training. Atlantic FICSIT Group. *Journal of the American Geriatrics Society.* 1996: 44(5):489-497.

 Authors' conclusions: Tai Chi decreased blood pressure, decreased fear of falling and decreased occurrence of falls.

Vellas BJ, et al. Fear of falling and restriction of mobility in elderly fallers. *Age and Ageing Journal of British Geriatrics Society.* 1997;26:189-193.

 Author's conclusion: The study indicated that about one-third of elderly people develop a fear of falling after an incident fall and this issue should be specifically addressed in any rehabilitation program.

###

To order additional copies of the books go to

www.fallpreventionadvisors.com or call
Infinity Publishing 1 877 289-2665